GRIEF

5 Lives-5 Stories-1 Need
Acceptance

SHANNON STEWART

Copyright 2018 by Shannon Stewart

2MCH4YA Global Entertainment

This is a work of fiction. Names, characters, places, and incidents are either products of the author's imagination or, if real, are used fictitiously.

All copyright, trademarks (registered or unregistered including without limitation the following marks: "Grief, 5 lives, 5 stories, 1 need…acceptance"), trade and business names, trade secrets, know-how and all other intellectual property rights in the book and its content (including without limitation the book design, text, and graphics connected with the book) are owned by or licensed to 2MCH4YA Global Entertainment/Shannon Stewart or otherwise used by 2MCH4YA Global Entertainment as permitted by law.

All rights reserved. No part of this book may be reproduced or transmitted in any form or by any means, electronic or mechanical, without written permission from the author, except for the use of brief quotations in a review.

Images licensed or owned by 2MCH4YA Global Entertainment

The content of book, including text, graphics, and images ("Content"), is educational only and not intended to be a substitute for medical advice, diagnosis or treatment. Although the health Content is reviewed and approved by health care professionals, 2MCH4YA Global Entertainment, Shannon Stewart, and the Health Care Professionals associated, do not guarantee the accuracy, adequacy or completeness of any information and are not responsible for any errors or omissions or for the results obtained from the use of such information. Always seek the advice of your personal physician or other licensed health care provider with any questions you may have regarding medical advice, a medical condition, or symptom. Never disregard, avoid or delay obtaining medical advice from your licensed health care provider because of something you have read in this book.

If you believe you may have a medical emergency, call 911 immediately. Any mention of products or services in this book is not meant as a guarantee, endorsement or recommendation of the products services or companies. Reliance on any information provided in this book is solely at your own risk. Please discuss any options with your licensed health care provider.

Published in the United States of America

Acknowledgements

I would first like to thank my Lord and Savior Jesus Christ through whom all things are possible. This book would not have been possible without the love and support of my husband Willie Stewart. I want to dedicate my very first novel to my mother, Ruby Marish. You instilled in me, good manners, self-esteem, and a love of family. You have been one of my biggest cheerleaders and gave me encouragement in every aspect of my life. I want to make sure that, as the world discovers me and my writing, they remember my sister Jaqueline Cummings and my father Michael Marish. Not a day goes by that I don't remember the way Jackie yelled to keep everybody in line as she cooked and the love she showed for her family, kids, and community. No holiday is the same without Michael and his barbecue and words of wisdom he passed on constantly. You both left us too soon and will never be forgotten. I also want to acknowledge all of my other siblings for their past and continued support as awesome brothers and sisters. "My birthday twin" Sharon Warren, "My ride or die" Lorrie Davis, Tamiko Madison, Shayla Reeves, Dwayne Dubose, Thomas Dubose, and Terreance Dubose. Shout out to all my nieces, nephews, friends, co-workers and everyone else not mentioned specifically here. I appreciate you and I get inspiration for every word I write from you guys being in my life.

Table of Contents

Chapter One:- Denial 1

Chapter Two:- Anger 8

Chapter Three:- Bargaining 15

Chapter Four:- Depression 23

Chapter Five:- Acceptance 30

Chapter One: Denial

Jackie pressed closer into Franklin's side. She didn't notice that he pulled away each time she did so. "You have to get closer. You don't want just half of your face in the picture."

"This seat is small."

"Then come toward me."

"It's hot." He slid his arm from around her, settling for laying it across her shoulders. Just before the camera flashed, he allowed it to slide off.

Climbing over him, her elbow knocked him in the jaw. Her apologies were half hearted, the excitement of seeing the photos making it seem as if she didn't even care. Anxious, she ripped the photos out of the cubby, tearing off the top left corner. Her face fell. She waved him over after he exited. Holding out the photos at arm's length, she turned them counterclockwise, stepping in and out of the light in attempt to get a better angle. After staring at it for several seconds, she snapped her fingers. "I know what it is."

"What?"

"You're not smiling."

"I never smile."

She cocked her head with a raised eyebrow. "You act like that's a good thing." Fluffing her hair, she used the booth's shiny, mirror like, chrome edging to apply a fresh layer of lipstick. "Come on. Let's take it again."

"I'm tired."

"Tired from what," she said. Jackie crossed her arms over her chest and jutted one of her hips out. "We ain't even been here that long."

Franklin rolled his eyes.

Grief

"You're mad because I wanna commemorate the day."

"You don't even know what that means." She tugged his hand. "Please baby. We can go after this. I promise." She put her lips next to his ear. "And I'll do that thing you like when I get home."

He turned his face to the side. "You don't have to."

"I like when you play hard to get."

Remaining stoic was getting harder by the second. He clenched his fists, which helped to diffuse some of his anger. The pain in his knee was beginning to descend toward his ankle. It was going to rain. He wasn't even supposed to be so active after surgery. But 'he promised'. "Let's just take the picture." He led the way into the booth.

Again, she sat next to him. She hopped into his lap just before the camera flashed.

He hid his grimace in his shoulder. His face remained like stone for the next three flashes. On the final one, he managed to conjure a sarcastic smile.

Jackie bolted from the booth. She was pouring over the pictures when he came out. Her smile was indicative of satisfaction. She slid them into her purse without letting him see. "Thanks baby." Standing on the tips of her toes, she pressed her lips into his cheek. "You're the best." The fact that he'd rather her hold onto his bicep than his hand was interpreted as an act of chivalry. She managed to convince herself that holding hands was childish, despite seeing the majority of other couples that were out choosing the same method to display their affections.

Franklin was working, which gave Jackie the house to herself. She invited over her best friend, Yandy for a night of drinking and binging on ice cream and Love and Hip Hop. They were six episodes in, having gotten through a large tub of ice cream.

Jackie sucked the ice cream off her spoon, using it to point out one of the girls that she wasn't particularly fond of. "Her man keeps dogging her. How many times did she catch him cheating?"

"Too many." Yandy scooped up the last bit of ice cream before resting the tub in the middle of the ottoman. She stretched before standing. "What flavor now?"

"Coffee. I don't get it Yan, why does she keep going back to him." She stared at the girl as if she was in the living room. "It's clear he don't want you sis."

Yandy swallowed her chuckle. The truth choked her. She had wanted to tell Jackie the truth for so long, but having been her friend since they were in elementary school; she knew how Jackie reacted to anything negative about her boyfriends. Over the length of Jackie's and Franklin four year relationship, what started as pity had transformed into mocking. The longer she thought about how people talked behind her back and what they said when she wasn't around, the more the pity returned. Her eyes vacillated back and forth from the girl on the screen to Jackie. Soon, she wasn't able to tell the difference between them. The truth caused the tip of her tongue to burn, but she swallowed it, feeling her stomach acid splash.

"You get lost," Jackie said with a laugh.

She pulled the ice cream out, using her hip to close the door. Sitting a bowl next to it, she warmed the spoon under hot water. "Just getting me some before you hog the tub." She laughed as Jackie's mouth dropped open.

"The disrespect."

"I'm just saying. You eat 70% of the tub. It's cool. I accept that when we're eating ice cream together that I'll only get a little bit." Entering the living room, she fell next to her. "That's why I don't call you when I have a break up."

"No. That's because you break up with a guy every other week. I'd be 300 pounds fooling around with you."

"That's alright," Yandy said, jabbing her side with her elbow. "Your shade ain't enough for my shine."

Jackie grew quiet, her concentration back on the show. The girl and guy, Teairra Marí and Akbar, were having another argument. She popped up at the studio and caught him with a girl sitting in his lap. He was doing the typical man thing – blaming her for not trusting him. She threw her spoon down in disgust. "I'm tired of watching this. It's the same old thing. The girls let the guys run all over them trying to be a 'ride or die'."

Grief

Yandy was unable to take it anymore. The secret on her tongue was threatening to burn a hole in the roof of her mouth. Having dealt with and lost many female friends like this before, she found that the best way to deliver the truth was to do so in a way that allowed them to come to the conclusion themselves.

"I wish I would catch Franklin doing some stupid stuff like that."

"How's that going by the way? You and Franklin."

"We're amazing. Couldn't be any better." She hopped up, returning with her purse. Jackie took a moment to appreciate the happiness the photos captured. She caressed Franklin's face, smiling at the subtle grin. "I love him."

"Are you sure he's the best thing for you? I mean, don't you get lonely being here by yourself all the time?"

"I got used to it. And that's what I have you for."

"Yeah, but…"

"But what?" Jackie turned so that she was facing Yandy full on. "But what?"

"Maybe it's just my mind, but I need to know what my man is doing."

"Franklin's not doing anything. He goes to work and comes home." Jackie glanced at the TV. "We're not like them. We're not with each other for money. That's clearly not the case. You remember how it was when we first got together."

She very well did. Yandy had spent the majority of their conversations trying to convince her that Franklin, who didn't have a job or car at the time, wasn't worth the struggle. She lost her voice more than once attempting to remind her that it wasn't her job to fix a man, let alone support one. In fact, they had a falling out about it that resulted in them not speaking to or seeing one another more than a couple of months.

She was determined not to let the same thing happen. The first time she failed to protect Jackie. She wouldn't let history repeat itself. This was no time to beat around the bush.

"I'm starting to think you know something I don't," Jackie said with a chuckle.

Yandy took a breath in and out. She set her spoon down. "Franklin doesn't love you. He doesn't even like you."

"Stop playing. That's a good joke girl. I know you don't like him, but –

"It's not about me not liking him. I'm trying to protect you. You need to break up with him."

Jackie scoffed. Scooting away from Yandy, her hip landed on the remote. The volume increased, the argument on the screen coming to life.

"You're just hating because you ain't got your own man," Teairra Marí said.

"Maybe that's why I can see that he's dogging you and has been since you started dating. You're just blind and in denial."

"Ain't nobody in denial. I know my man. He loves me and I love him."

Jackie let out a sarcastic snicker, peering at Yandy out the corner of her eye. "You could've written this episode." She slapped the lid back on the ice cream and put it back in the freezer. She remained standing, leaning against the island. "I can't believe you. I thought you were my best friend."

"I am your best friend."

"Then why are you trying to break me and Franklin up. We're happy. I'm happy. You're supposed to be happy for me."

"I can't be happy when he's running around behind your back," Yandy said. "It's my job to protect you from that." The weight lifted from her shoulders as she continued speaking. Her mouth was a faucet that couldn't, wouldn't be turned off. She spoke of all the rumors, about all the women that had come to her with stories about sleeping with him.

There was Brenda. Lacy. Courtney. Miranda. All girls that they knew and were friends with at one point or another.

"Where's your evidence," Jackie said.

Grief

"We get our phones mixed up a lot, so I decided to delete the texts. I didn't want you to find them."

On the TV Teairra Marí was sitting across from her former friend, both of them nursing a glass of wine. Teairra Marí, rolled her eyes each time the girl spoke, huffing and puffing each time she provided some compelling information. Without warning, Teairra Marí flipped the table and launched herself at the girl. The two rolled back and forth on the ground, the other patrons watching in horror. Security finally intervened, but not after clothes had been ripped and wigs and weave had been snatched. Teairra Marí, walking backward toward the exit, managed to outmaneuver the security guard, grabbing a glass and hurling the liquid in the others girl's direction. It was a direct hit. Three replays followed, showing different angles as if it was a football game.

"You're just jealous. You and all those other females. Can't stand to see no one else happy."

The girl assured everyone that she was okay. "Some people can't handle the truth. No good deed," she said with a laugh, patting her face dry.

Jackie's knee bumped into Yandy's thigh as she reached over her to retrieve the remote, muting the TV. She returned to her spot, folding her arms across her chest as she leaned against the counter. "So you don't have any evidence? You just have stories from a bunch of hoes that want my man."

"I have evidence."

"Show me."

Yandy's shoulders rose and fell. Her eyes begged for Jackie to believe her. They were answered with scorn. She pulled her purse into her lap and rummaged through its content. Pulling out a small envelope, she rested it in her lap and sat the purse aside. "You notice how me and Franklin have been getting along lately?"

"Yeah. Too bad you're pulling this crap now. He's not gonna want to have anything to do with you when I tell him."

Yandy removed the contents from the envelope. She put her shoes and socks on before slipping into her jacket. Removing her keys from her purse, she hugged Jackie. The embrace felt as if it would be their last. She left the strip on the counter. A hand on the doorknob, she looked back. "I'm sorry." She exited.

Jackie allowed a few seconds to pass before she dropped her eyes. Her stomach knotted, her mouthwatering. Flipping the strip over, tears burned her eyes.

The pictures captured Franklin with a full smile, happier than he had ever been. The face he smiled at was familiar. That face had just left.

Often times we figure out a situation and the trauma of figuring it out puts us on a grieving pathway. Many times that first stage, denial, is what surfaces. Rather than showcase how we respond to a loss of a loved one, I showed an example of the loss of a treasured relationship. All of the signs were likely right there. However, Jackie chose to deny the reality of the situation. "This isn't happening, this can't be happening," people often think. Denial is a defense mechanism that buffers the immediate shock of the loss. We block out the words and hide from the facts. This is a temporary response that should carry us through the first wave of pain or loss. Kübler-Ross and Kessler explain that being "in denial" doesn't mean that you aren't aware of the reality of the situation. It means that your psyche shuts down because you simply cannot fathom the enormity of the loss and aren't ready to deal with it. So when people say comments like, "I can't believe he's dead," it does not mean that they literally don't know that their loved one has died. It means that they are still paralyzed with shock and that the reality is too much for their psyche to handle. "Denial and shock help us to cope and make survival possible. Denial helps us to pace our feelings of grief." "As you accept the reality of the loss and start to ask yourself questions, you are unknowingly beginning the healing process." "You are becoming stronger, and the denial is beginning to fade. But as you proceed, all the feelings you were denying begin to surface." You can ultimately progress and grow, or forever be stuck in this stage of grief.

Chapter Two: Anger

Tyler caught the pass just like he had been taught – all hands, no body. Bracing himself, his body absorbed the linebacker's hit. He withstood the impact with the ground. The ball remained steadied. He had learned from his previous mistake of letting it touch the ground.

"First down," the official said.

In the huddle, everyone looked to the quarterback, Mitchell. There were 20 seconds left in the game. Enough for two plays. This was the moment he trained his entire life for. All the early morning workouts and the three-a-days. All the injuries, two shoulder surgeries, a broken arm, and more broken fingers than he could count. All the time watching film, memorizing defensive tendencies, staying so late that he went to class with only half an hour of sleep.

This was his time.

He was the last to break the huddle, the first to the line. He knew the route like the back of his hand. Taking a deep breath and closing his eyes, the image became clear. Jab with the right foot, sprint twenty yards, stop on a dime, keep the toes down while completing the catch.

He and Mitchell made eye contact. His nod was slight.

Mitchell pointed out the rushers and adjusted his protection. "Blue 16. Blue 16. Set. Hut."

Tyler's body took over.

Jab with the right foot, sprint twenty yards, stop on a dime, keep the toes down while completing the catch.

"Get back to the line," he said, waving his arms. "Get back to the line."

Mitchell stopped the clock with seven seconds left. Everyone gathered around him. "Alright boys. This is for the championship.

We've been practicing all year for this." He looked at Tyler, grabbing his shoulder. "I'm coming to you."

On the line, the 25 yards he needed to score never looked so far. He clenched and relaxed his hands to keep them from shaking. Breathing through his nose helped to calm the jitters in his stomach. As his mind settled in, he didn't see the cornerback lined up across from him. It wouldn't have mattered if he did, he wouldn't be denied. He had been waiting for the moment for far too long to let it slip through his fingers. Using his peripheral vision, he watched Mitchell point out different players, alerting the offensive line to potential rushers.

Just hold for three seconds.

"Red 19. Red 19. Set. Hut."

Tyler's foot slipped. Keeping his balance, he managed to out maneuver the cornerback. Running full speed, he was at the ten yard line when he saw Mitchell winding up. The shaking was gone from his hand. The ball left Mitchell's hands just as he was coming out of his break. It appeared to be moving at light speed. It thumped against his chest.

"He's at the five," the announcer said. "I think he's gonna make it! There's a defender barreling down on him. He's in the air..."

The air rushed through Tyler's face mask. He watched the thick white line glide underneath him. His bliss disappeared as his trajectory suddenly change. Unable to get his hands down, his shoulder broke his fall. He managed to roll over onto his back. He smiled to himself as he watched the people in the crowd high fiving, pumping their fists, and hugging one another.

"Touchdown Alabama! Say hello to your new national champions!"

His teammates lifted him to his feet before throwing him on their shoulders. Their excitement dulled the pain in his shoulder. As they lifted him up and down, he was able to ignore the heaviness pulling on his legs.

A week had passed since the championship game, meaning, it was time to get back to work. He had declared for the NFL Draft. His performance caused him to vault up the boards, citing him as the

Grief

number two receiver prospect.

Tyler, feeling the sun, burst into a seated position. Checking the time, he threw the sheets back. A moment later, his mom, Janet, walked into his room.

"I turned it off. You deserve to rest." She set the tray of food she was carrying at the foot of the bed, sitting next to it. She ruffled his hair, smiling at his smile. "How'd you sleep?"

"Pretty good. Dreamed about the game again." He patted the bed and looked through his drawers. "Where's my phone?"

"I have it. You wouldn't believe how many people called."

"Gotta start getting ready for the draft. No days off."

"Except for today," she said. "I feel like I haven't spent any time with you. How about a mommy-son date?"

"As long as you don't call it a mommy-son date."

"You're paying," she said over her shoulder as she left the room.

"I'm getting ready." Tyler fell back into the pillows, running through the victory as he had done every morning since. After a few minutes, he sat back up. Attempting to swing his legs out, he found that he couldn't. He tried again. Throwing the sheets on the floor, he tried a third time. Pulling each leg to the edge of the bed, he straightened his arm, lifting his bottom off the bed. He pushed himself to his feet. Remaining up right for a second or two, he felt himself beginning to lean forward. The ground knocked the wind out of his chest.

"What was that," his mom said.

"I can't feel my legs."

"What?"

"I can't feel my legs," Tyler said. "I can't feel my legs. I can't feel my legs."

"Stop joking Tyler."

"I'm not fucking joking. I can't feel my legs." Tyler tried to push himself up, only his upper body leaving the ground. He tried again. Tears began to stream from his eyes. He choked on his words as his mind did his best to process what was going on. The carpet caused his cheek to itch. He forced himself to think positive thoughts as his mom did her best to control her panic.

"The test is simple," Dr. Gauge said. "I'm going to poke at your legs and feet. All you have to do is tell me if you feel anything. Easy right?"

"Right." Tyler stared at the ceiling.

Dr. Gauge dropped his pen down the inside of Tyler's thigh. Not getting any reaction, he dragged it on top of his leg. He did the same on the bottom of Tyler's foot, still nothing. He said nothing as he looked at Janet.

"I'm ready."

"I'm done with the test."

Tyler looked from Dr. Gauge to his mom. "What?"

He tried to sit up.

"Tyler, honey, please calm down."

"I'm not paralyzed. I was walking all day before," he said. "I'm not paralyzed." He tried to slide his legs to the edge of the bed, neither of them budging. "I'm not paralyzed. The draft's coming up. I gotta get ready."

Dr. Gauge placed a hand on his shoulder. "Take some breaths. I'll come back to explain."

"Explain what? I can't move my fucking legs."

"Tyler."

"It's okay. It's a hard thing to process. You have delayed onset paralysis. You most likely have a vertebral fracture."

"Can I still play ball?"

"Depends on how surgery goes."

"Will he be able to walk again," Janet asked.

"From my previous experience, he should be able to walk

Grief

again with physical therapy. You're still under the university's insurance. I can schedule the surgery as soon as you're available."

"Schedule it for tomorrow," Tyler said. Alone, he laid back down, his eyes went to the ceiling. Gripping the sheets, tears slipped through his eyelids. He pressed his teeth together as he focused all of his mental faculties on moving. "Come on." The tears grew. "Come on. Please." His body remained still.

Five Years Later

Tyler hobbled to his chair, the leather stretching and twisting as it molded to his shape. Reclining and lifting his feet helped to relieve the pressure in his lower back. Turning the TV on, he scrolled through the guide, skipping over the NFL games. He turned on Days of Our Lives.

"Can we watch the Cowboys," his wife, Monica asked. "We have a bet going on at work."

"I hope you bet your money."

"It's not for money."

"Then you're not losing anything. No need to watch the game," he said. "Get me a beer."

"What's wrong with your legs?" She pinched the bridge of her nose. "I didn't mean that." Going into the kitchen, she twisted the cap off the bottle and handed it to him. "Can we please watch the game? I'll go to a bar next time."

"Why can't you go to a bar this time?"

"Don't feel like it."

"I don't feel like watching the game, so we're even."

"Any other guy would be happy to watch the game with me," she said. "Sometimes I swear I don't know why you're with me."

"Stop being so dramatic. Me not wanting to watch the game has nothing to do with you." He snatched the remote after she reached for it. "I'm not watching the game. Go in the bedroom if you wanna watch it."

"What the hell is wrong with you? We used to watch football

together all the time."

"The game is different. Softer. I don't like it."

"You're turning into a bitter old man. You hobble around here with a scowl on your face like the world did you wrong. News flash Tyler, you're still alive. Moping around isn't gonna change anything. I know what it's like to lose something you love, but –"

"You know what it's like?"

"Yeah, I know what it's like. I wanted to be a writer, but I had to give it up so I could support myself and you."

Tyler's heels thumped on the ground. He turned the TV off and leaned forward. His anger bubbled in his stomach, slowing crawling up his throat. "You gave up a dream? You don't have the discipline to write a book. I had my dream!" He showed her his palms. "In my hands! I was gonna be a first round draft pick! I was gonna be set for the rest of my life! My mom, who has been working for all her life, could have finally retired!" He grimaced as he pulled himself to his feet. Various joints and bones popped as he straightened his spine. "I didn't give up my dream. It was taken from me. We are not the same."

She shrunk away from him as he lowered her face to him. "Tyler, you're scaring me." She glanced at each of his arms, which was framing her head. "Please calm down."

"Calm down? You walk around here thinking you're better than me. Because you can walk faster than me. Because your legs work better. You're not better than me."

"I never said I was better than you."

"You didn't have to. It's in everything you do. You look down your nose at me when I'm the one in pain. When I'm the one that can't sleep more than a couple of hours at a time. When I'm the one that has to pop seven pills every fucking day just to feel normal and be able to function."

Their foreheads were pressed together. He matched her each time she moved, not allowing her to escape. His anger, just underneath the surface, made his skin red.

Tyler stood up, his chest heaving. He turned the TV back on.

Grief

"You want to know why I don't like watching football?" He tossed the remote in her lap. "It's because it should be me on that field. It should be my name that all those people are cheering. Now the only person calling my name is you." He staggered to the front door, where he grabbed his jacket and keys. "Enjoy the game."

This stage of grief is where we search for blame, feel intense guilt, and lash out.

As the numbing effects of the denial stage of grief begins to wear off, the pain of loss starts to firmly take hold. However, some people start immediately in the anger stage of grief. Tyler may have appeared to go directly into the anger stage, but he did deny his injury initially. When you can't deal with the reality of the situation, intense pain and loss can be expressed as anger. Your anger may be directed at your dying or deceased loved one or it could be directed at those who love and care for you. Your anger could be aimed at complete strangers, friends or family, the doctor who diagnosed the illness and was unable to cure the disease, or even inanimate objects like the walls we often see in reality shows with a fresh fist shaped hole in them. If you believe in God you may also become angry with God for taking your loved one from you and for not sparing your loved one and you from suffering. You may have been expecting God to prevent your crisis because you prayed and it still happened so you become angry. It is not uncommon for grieving people to go through a spiritual crisis. There is no limit to the depth of your anger or to whom or what it may be directed. Kübler-Ross and Kessler explain: "Anger doesn't have to be logical or valid." "It is important to remember that the anger surfaces once you are feeling safe enough to know you will probably survive whatever comes." Anger is usually at forefront of a barrage of feelings of sadness, panic, hurt, loss, and loneliness as you grieve. It is completely ok to be angry. "The more you truly feel it, the more it will begin to dissipate and the more you will heal." The stages are not linear. They can happen in any order.

Chapter Three: Bargaining

Nico flipped the gun over in his hands. He hoped his face didn't show his fear. Every night he practiced his poker face, but in the moment it felt like he hadn't practiced enough. He felt naked, the only one not wearing a mask. Being the newest, youngest, and smallest, he dared not ask for one.

"Don't look so scared."

"I ain't scared."

"Then stop looking like it."

"Chill out Gator. It's his first time," Reggie said. "You gotta go slow." He took the gun. He showed him a small button on the left side of the trigger. "Press this – the slide fell into his hand – to reload." He slammed it back into place and flipped a switch up and down. "That's the safety. If you're not shooting, keep it on."

"Stop babying him. He wanted in this shit, let him get his hands dirty."

"I don't want him to get hurt."

"He knows what could happen," Gator said. "He does his job right we'll all get out with the money and the drugs." His grip was heavy on Nico's shoulder. "You want the money don't you?"

"Ye-yeah."

"Then we good? You know what you're supposed to do right?"

"Keep everybody still," Nico said.

A car pulled into the driveway. "Ride's here. Let's go." Reggie grabbed Nico's arm before he walked out of the door. "Stay calm and this'll go smooth." He flipped the switch on his gun. "Safety on."

With it being a Friday the bank was more crowded than usual. The van pulled around back, lingering in the spot just long enough to

Grief

let the crew out. Nico was the last one out, taking a final look at the driver, who nodded at him. Closing the door, he jogged to catch up to the rest of the men.

Reggie opened the door, allowing the others to rush in.

"Nobody move. Get on your knees, take your cell phone and keys from your pockets. Everybody come from around the corner." Gator waved his rifle back and forth, causing everyone to squeal and hide their faces. Picking one of the tellers up by his collar. "Unlock the safe." He kicked him in the butt as motivation to get him to move faster.

"Keep control of them Nico," Reggie said, "I'm gonna help Gator with the money."

Nico's hands shook, his arms feeling heavier than they ever had as he extended them out in front of him. His mask suddenly felt too tight. He wiggled his nose to relieve the itch. He swung the gun to the left. "Don't move."

"Please. I have two kids."

His eyes fell to her hands, which were holding her swollen stomach. "Just stay still. This'll be over in a minute. I'm not gonna hurt you."

"No please." The teller slid across the floor. "I wasn't trying to – Gator's boot knocked his head back.

Gator delivered a hard right hook and kicked the man in the stomach. "You thought I wasn't paying attention. Huh?" He punched the man again. Wrapping his hand around his neck, he pressed the gun into the man's chest. "Since the cops are already on the way, I might as well shoot you huh."

"No, please. I didn't mean –

"I'll watch over them." Gator made his way into the center of the room. "Go help with the money."

Nico didn't move.

"You nigga. The safe." He waited until Nico had disappeared. "Ima tell you a little story about team work."

Setting eyes on the stacks of money, Nico's first instinct was to throw up. His stomach quivered as he stepped inside. It wasn't until the bag hit his chest that he acknowledged Reggie's presence.

"When you're done with that one, grab another one. We only have a couple of minutes before the cops show up."

His feet dragged as he started for the wall. With so much cash available to him, he didn't know where to start. Gator's barking urged him on. As he began stuffing the bag, he couldn't shake the feeling that he was being watched. He also had a strange sense that it was almost too easy. Finishing the bag, he tossed it along with the others and started on another. The question of how much they would walk out with tickled the back of his throat, but he avoided asking, not wanting to seem like the rookie he was.

"Hurry up. Twelve is close."

The sirens made Nico's hand move at double their speed. He knocked over entire columns of cash, shoveling the loose bills into the bag.

"That's enough," Reggie said, "We gotta go."

"Didn't I tell you to stop moving?"

The pop was no louder than a fire cracker. The collective gasps of their hostages left no air for him to breathe. He stumbled forward after Reggie ran passed him.

"What the fuck?"

"I told that muthafucka not to move," Gator said. "He shouldn't na moved."

Nico heard his name, yet he was unable to respond. His name never sounded more foreign. It sounded as if it was being yelled from several 100s of yards away. His eyes fell to the gun. He looked toward the panicked whimpering patrons. The pleadings and begging made it real. He looked around, his eyes wide as if he were seeing things for the first time.

Reggie burst back into the room. He yanked him by his arm. "Come on."

"What about the money?"

"We got enough. We gotta get out of here."

Grief

Nico tripped over his feet. Nausea turned his stomach. Saliva flooded his mouth. Just as they reached the lobby, the front door swung open.

"Get down on the ground and put your hands behind your head."

He froze. Shock made his mind numb.

"Drop your weapon."

"Do it Nico," Reggie said.

Nico sat the gun at his feet.

"On your knees," the officer said.

He dropped to one knee, sliding his other foot behind him. As the arrival of several other officers, his arms jerked as he went to put his hands behind his head.

"Gun." The officers pointed their guns at Gator in unison. Their sounds as if they were sending a fallen comrade off to the kingdom in the sky."

Their bullets rushed through Gator's body as if it wasn't there. His body continued to tremble after the last passed through him. He remained on his knees for a few seconds before he fell to the floor. Blood pooled around him, finding the path of least resistance. The bank, a community institution for the past 50 years, had seen better days, it's foundation beginning to settle.

The officer who instructed him to get on his knees forced his face to the ground. Placing his knee on the back of Nico's neck, he showed no restraint as he cuffed his hands behind his back. Reggie's blood crept toward him. It was less than an inch away when the officer yanked Nico to his feet. "You wanted to be a thug. Now you get to go where they go. You better hit the weights as soon as you get in there. You're small. Easy prey."

Hands being cuffed to the table Nico couldn't scratch his ear. There was nothing in the room to keep his attention. Having to resort to counting the notches in the handcuffs lead him to believe that the experts were right about his generation being addicted to technology. His adolescent mind still hadn't processed the full extent of his situation despite being locked in the interrogation room for hours. But he was alive. Having been so close to death, he was thankful just to be breathing.

Just as he got his mind to settle, the door opened.

The suited man said nothing as he entered the room. He purposefully avoided looked at Nico as he laid a folder in the middle of the desk. With that, he left again. Another hour passed before there was any sign of him.

The door opened again.

The two toned walls were the first break in the grey that Nico was allowed.

"He'll break if he wants to go home," the detective said. "What's the under? Put me in for $500." He closed the door behind him. "Sorry about that." He tossed his apple into the air, taking a bite." He sat down, crossing one leg over the other. "My name is Detective John. But you can call me Stew. All my friends call me Stew." He continued chewing as he looked through the file. "Nico Lockett. 17, all A student, track star. What's wrong with you?"

"Huh?"

"I said what's wrong with you? Some girl called your Johnson small? You getting bullied or something?"

"No."

"No? Then why are you committing bank robberies that resulted in two people getting killed?"

Nico had no answer. The truth was that he had everything he could ever want, two loving parents, all the money he could want. Anyone would have willingly followed him. His friends would have done anything he asked.

"Are you gay?"

"What? No."

"Ah," Stew tapped his chin, "you're in it for the rush. I thought the other guy came up with this, but it's you. You put all of this together."

"No I didn't. Re…I was just a part of it."

Grief

"Don't be shy now. I know a man that's trying to make moves in the world when I see one. You planned this. That means you get to take the rap for those murders. One dead lady plus one dead man, you know what that equals right?"

"I didn't kill anybody."

"Two life terms. No parole." Stew took the last bite out of his apple and shot it into the trashcan. "Say goodbye to school. Say goodbye to your parents. I hope you're not a virgin because well, I'll leave that to your imagination."

"I didn't kill them."

"I don't believe you Nico." He stood. "There's really nothing you can say. Not only were there multiple witness, but even your so called pal Reggie said you were the main man. They did all the hard work for me."

"I swear to God I didn't kill those people." Nico slammed his fist into the desk, the reverberation flowing back into his arms. "I didn't even wanna be there."

"Did they force you?"

"No."

"Then you wanted to be there." Stew uncuffed him. "Get up."

"Where are we going?"

"Taking you to jail. You're being charged with two counts of first degree murder." He pushed him toward the door. "Come on."

"I didn't kill those people, I swear. I didn't kill them."

"I have witnesses."

"They're lying," Nico said. "I swear to God."

"23 hours of lock down a day in a cell that's smaller than a bathroom. For every second of that hour that you're out you can't even blink because that's too much time for someone to slit your throat. Someone that's out to prove that they're capable of making moves. Just. Like. You. How do you think your parents will react when they get that call that you were found in your cell? How do you think they'll react finding out that you killed yourself because you couldn't stand the quiet anymore?"

Nico saw his mother and father's face when he closed his eyes. Their pain became real, with a burn in his heart as the imagery flowed through his mind's eye. He imagined his mother on her knees, clutching the phone to her chest, his father unable to console her. Tears poured down his face.

"You better get your mind right because it's happening." Stew pulled his arm. "Let's go."

"I didn't kill those people. What do I have to do? Please, I didn't kill them."

Stew studied his face. "Point the finger at Reggie."

"I'll do anything else. Please. I'll leave this gang shit alone. I'll focus on school. I won't touch a girl. I won't lie to my parents. I won't pretend to be tough. Please, you gotta believe me. I didn't kill those people." Nico fell into the chair, crying into his hands. "Please. I didn't kill those people." When he looked up, Stew was standing over him.

"I'm sorry Nico, I can't change what happened. Use it as a lesson to make better choices in the future."

Nico, tears dried, raised his head, resigned to his fate, the bargaining that had worked for every other situation failing him. There was only one thing left to do.

Often times when we are faced with a painful loss….loss of a loved one, loss of a job, or like Nico's case, the imminent loss of freedom, we may try to make a secret deal with God or a higher power in an attempt to postpone the inevitable. In this case, Stew represents the higher power. Bargaining is the "What if…." stage of grief. "What if I devote the rest of my life, to God, to helping others?" The bargaining stage of grief provides temporary escape from one's pain and provides hope. This gives a person time to adjust to the reality of the situation. Kübler-Ross and Kessler state: "When we accept that they are going to die we may bargain that their death will be painless." "After a death, bargaining often moves from the past to the future." "We may bargain that we will see our loved ones again in heaven. "We may bargain and ask for a respite from illnesses in our family, or that no other tragedies visit our loved ones. Bargaining may provide temporary escape and hope, but it is a stage that we absolutely have to get through in order to heal

Grief

during grieving. Otherwise, you continue to live in a false reality in hopes that your pleas can effect change.

Chapter Four: Depression

Dr. Hunter sat across from Benny. Today, he didn't have his notebook, his chest pocket was empty. Pulling his arms out of his sleeve, he rested the jacket on the back of his chair. He always had an easy going face. Today something was different. He didn't have the usual concern in his eyes. Instead, there was no compassion, perhaps even amusement.

Per their usual routine, he permitted Benny to be the first to speak.

Benny knew the trick, though he was never quite able to resist it. Many minutes passed. Finally, his need to express the sorrow he was dealing with forced itself from his chest. "My life sucks."

"Why does your life suck?"

"Everybody around me is either sick or dying. I hate my job, but I can't quit because I like my apartment. I almost had sex yesterday, but…"

"But what," Dr. Hunter asked.

"I couldn't because she wanted me to take my shirt off."

This would've been a normal concern for anyone else, but Benny was a gymaholic. Throughout their two years of working together, Dr. Hunter had convinced him to start looking into bodybuilding competition, both as a way to improve his self esteem and make more money.

"Why didn't you want to take your shirt off?"

"Because I'm fat." Benny stood. After a breath, he pulled his shirt over his head, revealing his rock hard abs. He turned to the left and right. "See." He pinched his side, stretching his skin. "Fat." Maneuvering back into his shirt, he sat back down. "What's wrong with having sex with a shirt on?"

"Nothing."

Grief

"Then why did she keep asking me to take my shirt off?"

"She liked you," Dr. Hunter said with a chuckle. "She wanted to see you."

Benny's face tightened. His feet danced, his leg beginning to bounce. Though his mumbles were incoherent, his tone was clear. He was beating himself up for having missed another opportunity. The negative voice in his head was chastising him about being a 'scared sissy boy'. He slammed his fist into his palm.

"Talk. Express."

"I just want to be fixed. I'm tired of feeling like this."

"What do you feel like," Dr. Hunter asked.

"Like, like – he looked around the room for something to inspire the right word – like a shadow. A cloud. I'm just floating by. Sometimes I'm grey. Sometimes I'm white. Sometimes I'm black. No matter what, I'm heavy. The rain is holding me down."

"What's the rain Benny?"

He grew quiet. The various ticks in his body were indicative of the effort his mind was putting forth to come up with an answer. Many memories materialized, more of them capturing moments of failure – his championship game losing strikeout, his failure to close a $1,000,000 deal, showing up late to his grandfather's funeral. In his view, his life was nothing more than one big giant failure. He glanced at the hand that landed on his knee. He shook it off.

"Do you think your life would be different if it wasn't you living it?"

"Absolutely."

"What if you only changed your name? Would your life be different then?"

"Probably. Benjamin doesn't mean anything special," Benny said. "People don't even call me that unless they're made."

Dr. Hunter tapped his chin. After a while, he got up and went over to his desk. He moved some things around, finding a pen, he clipped it to his chest pocket. Walking to the library, he ran his fingers along the spines of the books, sneaking peeks at Benny every few seconds. Throughout their time together, he had come to recognize that Benny grew anxious when the attention wasn't on him. Noticing the subtle bounce in his leg, Dr. Hunter continued scanning the spines. Finally, he grabbed a pair of goggles from one of the shelves and returned to his seat.

"Would you wish your life on someone else?"

"Uh, I don't understand."

"Your life sucks right?"

"Yeah," Benny said.

"It's so bad that you've thought about harming yourself?"

Benny's chin dropped, his eyes falling to his shoes. He twirled his thumbs around one another. The light layer of sweat made his forehead glisten. "But I didn't try anything. I couldn't do that to my parents."

"Your parents," Dr. Hunter tapped his chin while tracing the frame of the goggles. "Would you do anything for your parents?"

"Of course."

"If they were dying, would you do anything to save them?"

"Yes, of course."

Dr. Hunter set the goggles on the table for him to see. "Would you give them your life, as much as it sucks and as bad as it is, if it meant that they could live longer?"

"Yes."

Dr. Hunter picked up the goggles. "Benny – he looked him in the eyes – like most people, you have the banal ability to pull negativity out of everything that happens to you. You said your life would be different if you were another person. These – he gestured to the goggles – will give you that opportunity. But there's a caveat." He retrieved another set of goggles. "You have to give your life to that person." After handing them one of the pairs, he slid the other over his eyes. "Let's trade places."

"I don't know about that."

"Don't think about it. Just do it. You want to live another

Grief

life. This is your opportunity."

Benny hesitated as he reached for the goggles. He stared at them for a long while. "Do we really have to do this?"

"What are you afraid of? That you might realize that there's some people who have it worse than you?"

Convinced and wanting to prove that no one had it worse than him, he slid the goggles over his eyes and reclined into the chair. Nothing happened right away. "Is there a button I'm supposed to push or something?" Not a second later, everything went dark.

Benny woke up in a bed that he didn't recognize. His head feeling as if it were going to split into two, he pushed his hands into his forehead. An unfamiliar woman was lying next to him, murmuring something about it was his turn. The pictures on the dresser helped him realize that the experiment had commenced. He listened to the baby's cooing coming from the adjacent room.

Throwing the covers back, the woman, his wife, urged him to hurry up, calling him an old man and making jokes about his knees.

"I'm going out with the girls tonight."

Not knowing whether he should be upset or not, he said, "Again?"

"I need a break from the baby. I need some money for a new outfit too." Without turning over, she reached behind her. Her hand remaining empty, she peered over her shoulder. "Money please."

"I'll give it to you later."

Sitting up, she scoffed. She stretched across the bed and removed his wallet from the side table and took out $300. She took another $100 out. "I'm paying for drinks."

The baby began wailing.

"Go get him before I shoot myself in the head. Geez, he cries nonstop." She covered her head with a pillow. "Go. Hurry up."

Benny staggered to the other room. Not knowing the baby's name, he referred to him as son. Never having held a baby before, he adjusted him until it felt right. Finding a book, he got comfortable in the oversized chair and began reading. Just as he was falling asleep, the baby began wailing once more.

"There's milk in the fridge."

On his way to the kitchen, he stepped over beer cans and balled up clothes. A line of trash circled around the kitchen island. There was a faint stench of rotting food. He set the baby in a high chair. Opening the refrigerator revealed the source of the smell. The bananas were black, their juice beginning to puddle beneath. He didn't trust the milk. Searching for a replacement, he stumbled upon a drawer filled with envelopes. Curiosity got the better of him as he opened the one on top. It was a bank statement for a purchase north of $30,000. The subsequent ones he pulled out followed in the same manner, the amounts varying, $10,000, $5,000, $25,000.

His wife stumbled into the room, rubbing her eyes. "Jesus Christ." She snatched the milk from the fridge. "All you gotta do is warm it up and give it to him. He can hold the bottle himself. I swear I gotta do everything."

"I think it's bad," he said.

"It's not bad. If he gets sick we'll take him to the doctor. Ain't that what health insurance is for?" Opening a beer, she gulped it down, leaving the empty can on the counter. "Shut him up Marcus. You don't want me to have to do it."

The baby cried harder.

"Nothing's going to happen to you buddy. Mommy's just tired." He sat on the couch and turned on the TV, keeping one eye on the show and the other on the innocence in his son's eyes.

Benny woke up with a start. Turning the alarm off and stretching, he realized he was alone. Once the remnants of his sleep released him, he found that there was something different about his surroundings. Pulling back the curtains allowed the sun to beam through the window. It wasn't as bright. In fact, everything seemed dull, muted. After checking on his son, he cleaned up, and had a quick breakfast. Thankfully, the name of the daycare was on the refrigerator.

He made it to his appointment five minutes before it was supposed to start. The reminder in his calendar supplied the client's name.

Grief

"Hi Dr. Hunter."

He grew excited, always wanting to be the person on the other side of the questions. "What's on your mind today Sheila?"

She showed him her wrist, fresh red gashes traveling across them. "I did it again."

Benny did his best to hide his shock, swallowing doing nothing to rid his mouth of the excess saliva. "What made you – he gulped hard – do that to yourself?"

"I felt out of control. I messed up a report and my boss yelled at me. I forgot to get the dog's food after work. I got a ticket for erratic driving. My husband rejected me again. He doesn't even hide that he's not attracted to me anymore."

Benny didn't say more than 10 words for the duration of their appointment. His hopes that things would get better were quickly dashed, the next three appointments were similar in darkness.

When the day was finally over, there was nothing he wanted to do more than hold his son.

Arriving home, his wife's car wasn't in the driveway. He knew something was wrong, the house too quiet when he entered. Searching the living room and bathroom, he coached himself to take a deep breathe, willing his mind to think positive. A quick peek in his bedroom showed that it was empty. He paused just outside his son's room. An ominous feeling overwhelming him. After a few minutes, he finally stepped inside. The crib was empty. All the drawers were opened, the clothes that remained were strewn about. He ripped his phone from his pocket and called his wife. It went straight to voicemail. Hanging up, he called again. Getting the same result. The voicemail answered his call each of the next five times he dialed her number.

Returning to the kitchen, he found a note.

You're not the father Grayson deserves. You're probably not his dad. We both deserve better than you and my friend is gonna give that to me. Don't try to call. I'll call you when we're settled so I can arrange for the rest of my stuff.

His tears dotted the counter, melting into the paper. The silence gave way to the whispers of his demons.

Vision blurry, mind cloudy, he stumbled back to his bedroom. Dropping to his knees, his fingers were numb as he reached under the bed. He pulled the case toward him. Opening the top, he stared at the pistol. His sobs choked him as he picked it up. His prayer was incomprehensible. He put it in his mouth.

Click.

It should be noted that the type of depression that Kübler-Ross and Kessler references in the 5 stages of grief does NOT have sustained functional impairment and is NOT accompanied by suicidal thoughts. If your depression is impacting your ability to cope with everyday life over a sustained period of time—or if you are experiencing suicidal thoughts—please consult your family physician or a mental health professional immediately. With that said, it is appropriate to note that depression may occur when reality really sinks in. During this stage of grief, intense sadness, decreased sleep, reduced appetite, and loss of motivation are common. Kübler-Ross and Kessler state: "After bargaining, our attention moves squarely into the present." "Empty feelings present themselves, and grief enters our lives on a deeper level, deeper than we ever imagined. The depressive stage of grief often times feels as though it will last forever. But it's important to understand that this depression is not a sign of mental illness. It is the appropriate response to a great loss. During this phase it is best to embrace it because it is natural. Cry when you have to cry. Mourn when you have to mourn. But keep living. Experiencing the depression and not avoiding it will help it to serve its purpose in your loss. You will get better and it may still come back from time to time, but knowing that's how grief works....Keep living.

Chapter Five: Acceptance

Kimberly laid her head on her grandfather, Robert's, chest. His heartbeat, strong and loud, belied his outward condition. She glanced up upon feeling him stir. "Am I too heavy?"

"Of course not sweetheart." He guided her head back down. "This bed just sucks. Why don't they get beds for regular sized people?" It was a funny statement coming from a man that stood 6'5". He continued squirming, holding her in place as he slid a pillow under his lower back. "Now if you had a big head like that dad of yours." They laughed together. "You know you didn't have to come see me today. Didn't you have practice?"

"Yeah, but Coach let me go early."

He kissed her forehead. "You're so talented. I wish I could come watch you."

She reached for her purse. "You can." Pulling out her phone, she played the video of her last game. Tears came to her eyes as she watched his smile widen.

It was a smile that she had come to associate with true happiness. While other people had a signature piece of jewelry, a signature phrase or reaction, Robert's smile was his signature. Every time she saw him, he was wearing it, without fail, even when he was in pain. And in recent months, he had been in pain a lot. She noticed it in spite of him giving his best effort to hide it. She did a better job of hiding her hurt. Kimberly hated seeing him in pain.

"How many points did you have," he asked, after the video went off.

"Guess."

"10."

"Higher."

"15."

She pumped her thumb into the air. "Nope."

"20."

"Keep going."

His eyes widened, his mouth dropping open. "I know you didn't score 30 points."

Her smile traveled across her face as she nodded. "With 9 assists and 6 rebounds. We won by one. I hit the game winning free throw."

His hug was strong. He held her so tight that she was able to feel his heart speed up. The monitor also relayed the change. "I am so proud of you. Now I really wish I coulda been there. I woulda had my sign and my airhorn."

"You can't bring airhorns to high school games Grandpa."

"Says who?"

She didn't have an answer.

"Exactly. I woulda blew every time the other team shot a free throw," he said with a chuckle. He let his head sink into the pillows. A tear fell from his eye as he stared at the ceiling. "You have no idea how much I miss watching you play. I miss coaching you too."

"You were a really good coach."

"I know. Way better than that coach you got now. What's his name again. Baron. Bruce."

"Barker. His name is Coach Barker," she said with a laugh. "He's pretty good."

She recalled her younger days, when he was healthy and was able to run around with her. He would demonstrate a move, putting her body in the right position when it was her turn. He didn't yell. He didn't have to. He always said that a coach that has to yelled is bad at giving instruction. He believed in positive reinforcement, giving her a high five or a pat on the back whenever she did right or wrong.

"How many turnovers," he asked.

"Huh?"

Grief

"How many turnovers did you have?"

"Three. But two of them weren't my fault. I gave perfect passes, but both of the girls dropped them," she explained. She knew what was coming.

"Know your personnel," they said in unison.

"I know, I know. But they were so wide open. Like so wide open Grandpa." She hopped up from the bed and demonstrated both plays, of course exaggerating how badly her teammates missed the pass.

"Your college coach isn't gonna want to hear any excuses. You're the point guard. That means you're the leader. You have to know who is capable of what at all times. You're responsible for the other nine players on the court."

"I know. I'll be better next game." Kimberly squeezed back into the bed, placing her ear on his heart. The thumps were her favorite lullaby, singing a song that only they could understand. She laughed as he began rapping Curtis Blow's "Basketball".

Basketball was the foundation of their bond. It was what they had most in common. Before she even knew what the game was about or could even comprehend what was going on, they were perched in front of a TV watching whatever game was on. He was the first one to put a ball in her hands. He brought her first hoop, a Fisher price goal. They would spend hours playing one on one.

She glanced at her shoes, reading his name over and over. Ever since she learned about his diagnosis, she wrote his name on every pair of shoes and dedicated every game to him. She traced the numbers on her jersey. 13. His number. She promised herself that she would wear that number for as long as she played. Her tears began to flow as she thought about him never being at another one of her games, how their eyes would no longer connect during the pledge of allegiance. His voice would no longer boom over everyone else's, telling the referee to 'keep their hands off her'.

She was unable to control her sobs, which caused her body to quake.

"Aww, baby girl," he held her tighter. "I'm not going nowhere." He didn't speak, keeping her close as he rubbed her back. He began to cry, knowing that she was being strong for him. "Let it out. Good girl."

Kimberly had been his pride and joy. He had been just as happy about her birth as his own children's. His heart was wrapped around her little finger the first time he laid eyes on her. She was his angel. She was his fountain of youth.

After the wave had passed, she wound her arms around his waist. "I'm gonna miss you."

"Miss me. Where am I going?"

"You know…"

"All I'm doing is losing this body. I'll still be here. Every time you feel something tickle your ear – he blew on her earlobe – that's me. Every time you don't feel like getting up early to go train, but you do anyway, that's me. The voice that tells you to take it to the hole when your jump shot isn't falling, that's me."

"But you're not gonna be at the games."

"You're absolutely right," he said, "I'm gonna be in the game with you. Let me up."

She held his hands as he hobbled out of the bed.

"Show me your jump shot."

Kimberly flicked her wrist.

"I didn't teach you to brick like that. Shoot it for real."

She put more effort into the second attempt.

He sucked on his fingertips. "Ooh, that's sweet. You see sweetheart, I taught you everything you know, so I'll be in every shot you take, every dribble and every pass." He grimaced as he dropped to one knee, pulling out his suitcase. Throwing it on the bed, he unzipped it. His smile was wide as he pulled out the miniature goal and ball. A few coughs rumbled his chest after he made it to his feet. "I'm okay. They don't clean good under there." He hooked the goal up on the door. After dribbling the ball for a bit, he tossed it to her. "Shoot for it."

"You can't be serious."

"I'm very serious."

Grief

"You know you can't beat me anymore Grandpa. You haven't been able to since I was in Jr. High."

"I had to build your confidence," he said with a wink.

"Oh, that's what you were doing. I appreciate that."

"You need to warm up?"

Kimberly sunk her first shot. "Nope, still hot from practice. You might wanna stretch though. I'm strong, but I don't know if I can get you back in the bed by myself if you pull something. And I wouldn't know how to explain that to the nurses."

"Oh you got jokes?" He opened a band aid and slapped it in the middle of her chest. "For your hurt feelings after I remind you who taught you everything you know."

She sank another shot. And another. "You do not want these problems Grandpa."

Robert twisted his spine and touched his toes. "Let's see what you can do with defense on you."

She tossed the ball to him. "Check."

He tossed it back. "My game to lose."

***

It was the day of the funeral, but Kimberly wasn't sad. Despite all the grief going on around her, she smiled. She half listened as the preacher spoke about what a great man Robert was and how he took every opportunity to brighten someone's day. After the choir sang, it was her turn to speak.

Waiting for the crowd to settle, she pulled out her notes. Having played in front of huge crowds, the multitude of faces staring back at her didn't make her nervous. "I'm Kimberly, Robert's granddaughter. No offense to my parents, but Grandpa was my favorite person in the world. He taught me how to play basketball. He's the reason why I love it so much. He's the reason why I'm so good."

She recalled numerous stories from her childhood – when they spent the night in the gym and her mom filed a missing person's report because they forgot to call her, the time he knocked her tooth out, catching her with an elbow, and the time she scored 60 points in a game.

"I was sad before because he wouldn't be at my games anymore," she said. "Anybody's whose been to my games knows how loud he was." Everybody laughed. "I was sad because I wouldn't be able to watch my film with him anymore. Most of all, I was sad because I was losing the best coach I ever had."

The preacher hugged her, her parents going up to the podium as she began to cry. Taking a moment to gather herself, she balled up the notes, using the paper to dab at her eyes.

"Me and Grandpa got to play one more game before he passed. And you'll never guess what happened."

"What," the crowd asked.

"He won."

Everyone began laughing and clapping, reminiscing about how good of a player he was.

"I'm not sad today because I remember what he told me. Grandpa told me that even though he wouldn't be able to watch me anymore, he would be in the game with me." She shot an imaginary jumper. "He's in every shot I take. He's in every dribble and pass. He's that voice in my ear telling me to keep going when I want to quit. He's the calming presence that reminds me to move on to the next play.

Grief

My grandpa isn't going anywhere." She stepped down to the floor and retrieved her purse. She removed her jersey, kissing the numbers before she rested it on the casket. Climbing back up the podium, she wiped her eyes. She kissed her fingertips and pointed to the sky. "I love you Grandpa. Now we can play together."

In this stage of grief, you have finally accepted the reality of a painful loss and that nothing will change that reality. Acceptance does NOT mean that you are "cool" or "indifferent" regarding loss. According to Kübler-Ross and Kessler "Most people don't ever feel okay or all right about the loss of a loved one or any sort of monumental loss." This stage is all about "ceding to the reality that a loss is very real and recognizing that this new reality is a permanent reality." Regardless of which stage you start in, or what order the stages occur in, getting to this final stage is important because adjustment occurs which can result in complete healing. "Kübler-Ross and Kessler's ground-breaking work on the 5 stages of grief changed the way that we think about bereavement. It also reassures us that there is no correct way or time to grieve, and encourages us to seek professional support if we get "stuck" in our grief. Kübler-Ross stressed that the concept of the five stages of grief should only be used as a tool to help us understand the emotions that we cycle through when we grieve. The 5 stages of grief don't define us. In fact, on her deathbed, Kübler-Ross wrote: "I know that the purpose of my life is more than these stages. "I have been married, had kids, then grandkids, written books, and traveled." "I have loved and lost, and I am so much more than five stages. And so are you." "It is not just about knowing the stages. "It is not just about the life lost, but also the life lived." One final thought…Acceptance is a process and not an end point. Did you notice any of the 5 stages in this final story or even more toward the end? Maybe there was a bit of denial as she ignored the preacher or others at the funeral? Maybe a tad bit of anger as she balled up her notes? Maybe some bargaining as she envisioned him still being here with her? Maybe some depression as she began to cry during her speech? "Finding acceptance may be just having more good days than bad." JUST LIVE.

PLEASE GIVE ME YOUR FEEDBACK

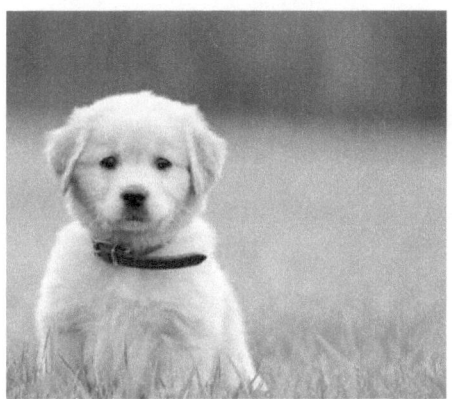

Your opinion matters and it helps other readers. I really appreciate you taking the next couple of minutes to review this book on amazon to help other readers. Please go to the following link to write a review. Thanks.

https://goo.gl/jZmknQ

www.ingramcontent.com/pod-product-compliance
Lightning Source LLC
Chambersburg PA
CBHW030541220526
45463CB00007B/2935